A Year of Meditations

Assembled by

Andy Gilbert

Copyright notice

Contents

A Year of Meditations

Why should you meditate?

The goal of meditation is to make our minds less cluttered and more focussed on what is important to us. The mind is an open book that the brain keeps filling with notes of what the detritus of our daily life is doing.
Think of it like when you watch a movie on TV. Your focussed mind is concentrating on the plot line. The unfocussed or peripheral edges of your mind are also taking in the fact the hero's computer is an 'Apple'. Or the phone he is using is three years out of date and you are so glad you upgraded yours to the galaxy S8 with the bigger memory chip. Now you can have your calendar sync direct to it, and that reminds you to check if your meeting tomorrow is at 9.30 or 10.30. Out of the corner of your eye you notice the cat is poking around at the edge of the book case. Don't tell me we have mice again. You have now had maybe a dozen side thoughts that have taken you away from the film you thought you were concentrating on. What the heck is happening in the film plot!
Life is like that.
We may be doing just one thing, but our brain will keep intruding with reminders and random

thoughts of every other facet of your life. Often that is a good thing as it keeps us organised on a broad level. It also helps us be alert to dangers.

Often it is a bad thing. We are reminded of all of the things that we have not done or should have done. That distracts us from what we should be focussing on. So that current focus is added to the list of things we have not done well and the pressure mounts on us.

Focus is a word we use to describe our total concentration on one thing. And it is probably the wrong word. We may be focussed on our career, but we also have to remember to do the weekly shopping and get the car serviced. Instead of using the word focus, let's use the term:

'Main area of concentration at this point in time'.
Alternatively let's use words like 'Here' and 'Now'.

Meditation allows you to let one thing be the 'main area of concentration at this point in time'. Other things may drift in and out of your mind, but the meditating mind will let you permit these things to drift on out of your 'here and now' awareness.

Let me repeat the opening line: "why should you meditate".

Because it allows the mind to relax by concentrating on only one thought. If you can decide what that thought is, beforehand, you will enjoy a peaceful, restful, relaxing twenty minutes or so. When you come out of your meditation your mind is totally relaxed and ready to take on anything your brain chooses to throw at it.

I could comfortably write an entire book on the benefits of meditation, but I won't. What I would like you to do at this point is try a simple meditation technique for ten minutes.

Sit back in a comfortable chair. Preferably an armchair.

Look around the room and pick out any object in the room. It may be a vase, or the TV, or the curtains. For this example, I'm going to use the TV.

Close your eyes. Think about the object in your mind's eye. Think about the shape of it. Be gentle and don't force the mind to remember everything you can recall. Just think about, gently, it for a minute. What shape is it? Have you ever noticed the curve of the frame as it nears the screen? How many little lights does it show when it is switched on?

At any time, something else may hover into your awareness. Let it come in and don't think about it. Allow it to drift on through your awareness and disappear.

What kind of stand is the TV on? What brand of TV? Is it a smart TV? Have you ever looked at all the ports on the side?

Sit and think/meditate about the TV for perhaps five minutes. Gently bring yourself back to the awakened state. Now look at the TV. You will now see it in a different light. Every curve in the TV was designed by a team of designers in Japan or Korea or wherever. They probably spent three months of their lives designing the shape of the box, so you would enjoy its visual appeal. How many millions of dollars went into developing the various extra features it will perform?

By thinking/meditating on the TV for just five minutes, you now have a different awareness of just what an incredible and aesthetically pleasing design it is. Yet you have been staring at it for the last few years and never even noticed most of the things you are now aware of.

Now, if you could take that simple technique and use it on aspects of your life, think how much more aware you would be of everything around you.

Meditation as a part of your daily life habits will bring you an immense amount of peace and focus. It allows you to walk away from all the petty things in your life and put them into some kind of perspective. It's free and it's freeing.

I strongly suggest that you give it a try. On a worst-case scenario, you may fall asleep and have a pleasant little doze. But on a best-case scenario..........................

Time for a new chapter. We'll look at some meditation techniques and practises

Chapter 2 meditation techniques

Posture

There are way too many meditation practitioners who would have you sitting cross-legged on a mountain top. Is it necessary? Not really, but it all adds to the mystique of the hermit-like existence of the individual who wants to be at one with the world.

Unfortunately, the world is not that interested in you. You are your own world. You are your own reality. (That's a great meditation all on its own). So, let's get organised on you doing what is comfortable to you.

I have a couple of favourite meditation postures and they work fine for me.

One is in a recliner type easy chair. Leg rest extended and the back support eased backwards a little. On the odd occasion I may doze off, but that only illustrates what a relaxed state I have achieved. My second favoured position is lying in bed. I lie on my back; my head rests on a comfortable pillow. Legs together and hands linked across my stomach. I am warm and comfortable and I feel very safe.

Whatever position you wish to adopt is fine. Meditation is a mental technique. It is not a test of physical agility or endurance.

Breathing.

Have your eyes closed and turn your attention to your breathing. Breathe normally, preferably through the nose, without trying to regulate your breathing pattern. Just get into a smooth breathing pattern. Within a minute your breathing will become shallower, as you relax. Be aware of the breaths entering and leaving your body. This consciously aligning yourself with your breathing helps to relax the whole body and starts to quiet your mind from other thoughts.
Initially other thoughts will come into your mind. Let them come in and drift on out again. If you ponder on them, they will take up some of your mind concentration. So, it is important to just let them go by. Keep your attention more aligned with the rhythm of the breathing.

Go somewhere safe.

Create a safe space in your mind. It may be in the middle of a field on a warm summer's day. Imagine how long the grass is. Feel the heat of the sun overhead. You feel safe and secure.
It may be in a woodland glade. You can see and feel the warmth of the sun as it dapples its way through the overhead branches. There is a gentle breeze

drifting through that is keeping you pleasantly cool. You feel safe and secure.

It may be on a lake. It may be an actual place from your past. Whatever you choose. Take yourself there, in your mind. When your breathing has slowed, and you feel you are inside the rhythm of your breathing. My safe space is on the edge of a forest, looking out over a green field. There is a wide stream flowing past me. I cannot see the stream, but I can hear its gentle rhythm.

Give (thanks) before you receive (insights).

This is not absolutely necessary but, for me, it is something I have always done. You are now in a peaceful place. Your head is in a peaceful space. Be thankful. You will more than likely come out of your meditation with energy and peace. If you meditated on a thought, you will more than likely receive some insights. So be grateful and give thanks to whatever deity you follow. If you don't have a deity, give thanks to the Universal force. It's a personal thing for me, but I feel I owe something to somebody or something for the gift of meditation.

Ponder on your idea.

I used to say think about 'something' but thinking always seemed to be too forced. I usually go into a meditation with something to think about, beforehand.

As an aside, I firmly believe we have two levels of awareness. Our lower level of awareness is what we have learned since we were born. If you like, it is how we survive the day to day life we are going through. I also believe we have a higher awareness. You can call it the universal force, which we can tap into. The knowledge of the ages, if you like. When I meditate I leave the lower level of awareness behind and relax in the flow of universal knowledge and higher thinking. It works for me and it works well. I try not to analyse my preplanned question or point-to-ponder. I only hold the thought in my awareness and wait to see if anything comes through to make me wonder about something.

Disturbances to your focus, or lack of focus.

Until you get a little more practised in your meditation, it's a given that random lower level thoughts will intrude upon your consciousness. I deal with them in two ways. If it just a random thought about, say, what is for lunch: I will allow the thought to enter without giving it any attention, usually it will just drift on by. If the thought is a negative thought, I push it toward the stream in my safe place and allow it to wash away downstream.

Whatever you think about that thought, it works for me.

Mantra (s)

A mantra is a sacred utterance, according to the sacred scripts. They are used in many religions as a prelude and focus to prayer of meditation. Many religions believe the 'word' has its own vibrations and spiritual powers. I don't totally fall into that category. The 'word' or Mantra used as a chant is a means of focussing the inner energy of the chanter. I have sat, and took part, in a meditation circle where a mantra was being used by a group of about twelve people. The chant seemed to take on an energy all its own. It almost seemed to form a vortex within the circle and lift us all. It was an amazing and uplifting experience that I have not felt since. The most common Mantra is the word "AUM" which is pronounced ORM in western tongues. For myself I use any two soft syllables in a soft rhythm if I feel the need for to use a Mantra to focus my mind.

Practise

If you want to get a better understanding of anything, you have to practise the skill. Meditation is no different. Now let's get on to the meditations

The meditation points I have selected are all pearls of wisdom, or proverbs, that have been passed down through the ages. Some of them do not readily sit with the society of today. All I ask you is that you meditate upon them and discover what they can say to you as an individual.

I have deliberately left a blank page opposite each thought. Use that page to write down your thoughts or revelations that may come to you. It will become a handy reference to your next days meditation and also something to look at when you pick up the book again, in a year or so's time.

As a last thought, I have always believed there is a greater force around us. Some may call it the Universal force or Spirit guides or even the God force. What ever you call it, I believe it is there to guide us. As an alternative to going through the book and meditating on one topic for a week and going to the next page, try this: just open the book at any page and perhaps the 'Universal force' will help you open the book at the page that is correct for you to think about today.

Chapter 3: A year of Meditations

I offer you a year of meditations in this book. But there is a catch. There are just 52 pages of sayings and they are each followed by a few thoughts of my own.

The reason for this is as follows. If you think back to when you learned your ABC's or your multiplication tables, you will remember that you learned them by repetition. I'd like to think that if you only meditated on a thought for one meditation, you would have some thoughts that you might find revealing to you. Perhaps something about your inner self or your lifestyle. If you do another meditation on the next topic on your next meditation session you will again get some inner revelations but you will quickly lose the thoughts you gained the previous day. I'd far prefer that you meditated today on whatever page you are up to. Tomorrow do it again. You will find that your first thoughts will quickly come back to you and you will also go down a further path on those thoughts.

Try and meditate for three days in a row and then take a break for a day. Meditate again for another two days and have another day off. You will quickly realise that your thoughts are becoming deeper and more revealing to you. Also, if you take the full week to meditate as I asked above, you will find the thoughts are becoming a part of your everyday thinking processes.

Enjoy the meditations.

Enjoy exploring your thoughts.

Enjoy your life!

Meditation 1

Firewood alone will not start a fire.

Think about his one in a personal context.
Will you be happy if you are fabulously rich, but have very poor health?
A great work life but a lousy home life. ?

Your thoughts and notes.

Meditation 2

The door to virtue is heavy and hard to push

What is this saying to you?
It is hard to be virtuous?
Or is it saying that a virtuous man cannot be pushed around?
What is it saying to you?
How does this apply to your life, today?

<u>*Your thoughts and notes.*</u>

Meditation 3

It is a waste of your time and energy to worry about losing your job. It would be far more useful to focus on getting another job or being better at your current job.

Stop worrying about what people think about you. Spend your energy on being with people who are much less shallow. You will end up with less worry and better friends. When you woke up this morning, you had so much energy to last you through the day. How much of it did you waste worrying about the things you have no control over?

<u>*Your thoughts and notes.*</u>

Meditation 4

One generation will plant a tree,
another generation sits in the shade.

What can you do to make the world a better place
for the next generation?
What mistakes did your parents' generation make
that are not helping people today? Are you going to
make the same mistakes?

<u>*Your thoughts and notes.*</u>

Meditation 5

Use your time wisely.
It will come to an end someday.

And we don't know when that time will come.
Use your time wisely.
What have you done today to make tomorrow better for you. And what will you do tomorrow?

<u>*Your thoughts and notes.*</u>

Meditation 6

You can't fill your belly painting pictures of bread.
If wishes were horses, beggars would ride.

John F. Kennedy said "Ask not what your country can do for you. Ask what you can do for your country".
 The world does not owe you anything, but what can you do for the world, YOUR world!

<u>*Your thoughts and notes.*</u>

Meditation 7

Do not tear down the East wall to repair the West wall.

Robbing Peter to Pay Paul?
Taking with one hand and giving it away with the other, just to try and keep your head above water?
What are you doing to increase your net worth?
More importantly, what are you doing to improve your perception of own self worth?

<u>*Your thoughts and notes.*</u>

Meditation: 8

Everything has a ripple effect.
Ask yourself this. Are you someone else's emperor?
Is there someone around you who shivers when you are angry? Do they deserve that?
Be more aware on how your actions may impact on others.
Be the calm eye of the storm. The gentleness where people feel safe before venturing once again into the storm that be all around, if we let it.

<u>*Your thoughts and notes.*</u>

Meditation: 9

Don't make the same mistakes others have already made.
 How many times have you gone ahead, foolishly, when a wiser person would have asked someone who had already travelled that path
Will you make that mistake again?

<u>*Your thoughts and notes.*</u>

Meditation :10

The wise men are not always those who speak loudest.
The loudest men are not always those who speak the wisest

Think Donald trump and his manner
Think of the Dalai lama and his way of doing things.
Who would you listen to for words of wisdom?
And where do you stand?

<u>*Your thoughts and notes.*</u>

Meditation: 11

Those who are carried on a throne are men.
Just like those who carry the throne.

All men are created equal. Some men feel a need to follow a leader and elevate him. Some men are their own leader.

And you?

<u>*Your thoughts and notes.*</u>

Meditation :12

Are we a body with a soul?
          Or are we a Soul with a body?
 Give your physical body a rest and meditate on this point.
 Is it the soul doing the thinking?

<u>*Your thoughts and notes.*</u>

Meditation :13

Think about what you are striving for
                    And why

<u>*Your thoughts and notes.*</u>

Meditation : 14

Is it saying 'don't walk around with your head in the
clouds?'
Is it saying, look at what the world has to offer you if
you take the right path?
What is it saying to you?

<u>*Your thoughts and notes.*</u>

Meditation : 15

The house with an old grandparent is a house with a jewel.

Our revered old folk have already trodden our path and made the mistakes that we are yet to make. Respect them and their wisdom.
Find some time to talk to an older person and listen to their story.

<u>*Your thoughts and notes.*</u>

Meditation : 16

You can lose your gold and be poor again
You cannot lose your learning and be ignorant again

<u>*Your thoughts and notes.*</u>

Meditation :17

Enough shovels of earth, a mountain.
Enough buckets of water, a river.

When you look around and see the state of our world and you are tempted to say, "But what can I do?" think of this meditation

<u>*Your thoughts and notes.*</u>

Meditation : 18

To succeed, consult three old people

The wisdom learned from yesterday will still be wise tomorrow.
 Do you know three old people?
And when did you last listen to them?

Your thoughts and notes.

Meditation : 19

I was told by a very wise man that no one is completely useless. Even if they only serve as a bad example, they have a value to us.
 Think of how that thought has affected your life.

**Your thoughts and notes.**

Meditation : 20

To understand your parents' love...............
...............bear your own child

Until you have walked in their shoes, you cannot understand them

<u>*Your thoughts and notes.*</u>

Meditation : 21

Many things mature with age. Cheese, Wine and Ginger are just a few,
 So do people!
Have you matured?
In what way?

<u>*Your thoughts and notes.*</u>

Meditation : 22

Don't rely on others when you can be better prepared, yourself.
Become self-reliant and you become more valuable.
More valuable to yourself and to the whole world.
Think about that concept.

<u>*Your thoughts and notes.*</u>

Meditation : 23

 This so simple.
And yet, still so profound

<u>*Your thoughts and notes.*</u>

Meditation : 24

The poor are too busy amassing pennies to worry about amassing dollars.
Which is wiser?
Can one learn from the other?

<u>*Your thoughts and notes.*</u>

Meditation : 25

Everyone dies.....................

.............................but not everyone lives.

What can you do today, to prove you are alive?
You only have to prove it to yourself.

<u>*Your thoughts and notes.*</u>

Meditation :26

Do not try and live forever...................
.... you will not succeed.

Try and live a little more for Today!

<u>*Your thoughts and notes.*</u>

Meditation :27

Fortune and flowers do not last forever.

Both need constant attention to thrive

<u>*Your thoughts and notes.*</u>

Meditation :28

The sun shines even after the worst storms.

Look up into the stormiest sky.
Beyond the darkest clouds that you can see, the sun
is still shining.
What is stopping you from seeing the sunlight?
And what can you do about it?

<u>*Your thoughts and notes.*</u>

Meditation :29

The world does not owe you anything.
 But remember what it has given to you.
Someone who smiled at you offered you the gift of happiness or even love.
Remember that time and count it as a small blessing

<u>*Your thoughts and notes.*</u>

Meditation : 30

- Zimbabwe native saying.

Always try to be the best you can be. Don't just exist, LIVE!
On a deeper level, remember this
Happiness and sadness are both a choice that you make. Why do you choose to be sad? Why not choose to sing?
Things happen to you. It's always your choice as to how you react!

<u>*Your thoughts and notes.*</u>

Meditation :31

Living and learning is like rowing upstream. You must advance or lose all.

If you are standing still you are being passed by others. Are you keeping up with others or are you happy to just watch them go by?

<u>*Your thoughts and notes.*</u>

Meditation : 32

Ideas never work unless you do.

Opportunities will never profit you. Unless you take hold of them and use them.
And some of my best ideas appear during my meditations.

<u>*Your thoughts and notes.*</u>

Meditation : 33

The meek shall inherit the Earth
The brave ones will live in the heavens.
The Holy books may not say it that way, but I have
always thought that this was what it meant.
What does it mean to you?

Your thoughts and notes.

Meditation :34

If you give no help to others.....
you are wasting those prayers to Buddha

Why should fortune favour you?
                    If you do not favour others.
What goes around comes around.
Reap as you shall sow.
Do as you would be done by.
In the Bible it is called the Golden Rule.
Maybe it could become a golden rule for you?

<u>*Your thoughts and notes.*</u>

Meditation :35

Many books do not use up words.
Many words do not use up thought

Another way of saying this is "That empty vessels make the most noise"
 Meditate today and be profound.
Look at what we hear from our nations leaders and wonder about the above meditation

<u>*Your thoughts and notes.*</u>

Meditation : 36

Your world needs leaders.

I'm actually talking about just your world. Are you leading yourself or are you being led around with no apparent direction.

How many generals are leading you in different directions?

Be in charge of your own destiny.

Be your own leader

Be your own general!

<u>*Your thoughts and notes.*</u>

Meditation :37

In life fear the judge,
                in death fear the devil.

Is there such a thing as a Devil?
Is there such a thing as heaven or paradise?
In life, the Judge whose opinion you hear the most often is your own self.
 I believe that if we all judged ourselves less harshly, then we would be too happy to worry about the devil.
Think about this in your meditation. The concept of a devil is something that was tossed into the Bible some 400 years after Jesus died. Why worry so much about something that is really only a postscript to a Judean - Christian history book.

<u>*Your thoughts and notes.*</u>

Meditation :38

A good teacher ...
.......is better than a barrow load of books

Do you remember back to your schooldays when there was that one teacher who could get you to work better than any other teacher you had met?
Compare that to the teacher who started every lesson with "Get your books out and read chapter 11..."
Who did you want to have as a teacher?
Are you teaching anyone? A work subordinate, perhaps?
Do they look forward to working with you?
How about your children?

Your thoughts and notes.

Meditation : 39

In addition to meditating on this thought, also meditate on this:-

Where is your mountaintop?

Do you have a mountain top you would like to climb? If you don't set some fairly clear goals, you will end up wandering around the base of the mountain looking up at the happy faces of all those who have reached their mountain top.

Think about it.

<u>*Your thoughts and notes.*</u>

Meditation : 40

Common-sense says you should have learned your lesson, the first time.
Another thought. A mistake with pain attached becomes a Lesson which we generally learn more from.
Why is that?

<u>*Your thoughts and notes.*</u>

Meditation : 41

I once had the privilege to meet a very famous Dutch artist in New Zealand. He had just arrived at the Airport. I asked him where his luggage was. He pointed to his shoulder sack." If it won't fit in here, I will not need it. I only carry what I actually need"
And the rest of us struggle around with all our baggage. Physically and literally!
If I can make this meditation really simple, I'd say jettison our excess baggage.
What 'baggage are you carrying around that you could relieve yourself of?

<u>*Your thoughts and notes.*</u>

Meditation 42

"If you're not happy, you can become happy. Happiness is a choice."

 In an earlier meditation we talked about choosing to be happy or sad.
 This might be slightly different way of saying it, but it's a point worth repeating, if a little more obviously.

<u>*Your thoughts and notes.*</u>

"Happiness comes from you. No one else can make you happy. Only you make you happy..."

I can't recall who said this but they had a great grasp on life. Whatever happens to you, it's always you who makes the decision to react and be happy or be sad.
It's your choice.
 Always, it's your choice!

<u>*Your thoughts and notes.*</u>

Meditation 44

I have met a lot of happy people in my life. Many of them had given up the struggle to conform to Society's norms and decided to be themselves and be happy.

The more we are ourselves, the more we attract similar people to ourselves and the better our life becomes.

Think about it. what are you repressing about yourself to conform and have friends that you really don't care too much about?

Your thoughts and notes.

Meditation 44

Happiness isn't a constant. You get fleeting glimpses of it and the rest of it, you're fighting for those moments and those moments are what make it all worth it".

 When you get to your mountaintop, you can't stay there. You have to come down again. How far you come down is up to you.
But until you have experienced the lows you will never truly realise the heights of happiness.
You can't be happy until you know Sad.
You can't love others until you love yourself.

<u>*Your thoughts and notes.*</u>

Meditation 45

You can only be happy at what makes YOU happy. If stamp collecting is your idea of happiness, then go for it!

If being a Lesbian does it for you, then be a lesbian!

Or if it's hang gliding or playing golf or going on overseas trips etc, then set yourself some 'you-time' to be happy. You deserve it.

<u>*Your thoughts and notes.*</u>

Meditation 46

A sure way to lose happiness, I found, is to want it at the expense of everything else."

Happiness is something that happens. Often you may make plans for it to happen. Sometimes it just happens when you hear a good story.
Realise the difference between the satisfaction of a plan coming together and the sheer enjoyment of being happy.
Think about that difference.

<u>*Your thoughts and notes.*</u>

Meditation 47

I agree wholeheartedly with this idea.
Sometimes you have to be stupid and selfish to really enjoy yourself.
Good health is a given.
Selfish? Totally, you have to allow yourself to be happy at the expense of other things, sometimes. It gives you spontaneous joy.
Stupidity? We spend so much time trying to conform to society that we seldom let our guard down because we think that is the wise thing to do.
Be stupid, sometimes it's so much more fun!

Your thoughts and notes.

Meditation 48

There may be Peace without Joy, and Joy without Peace, but the two combined make Happiness."

This another combination that defines Happiness. Think about the combination of Peace and Joy and imagine the more mellow sort of happiness you can achieve.

<u>*Your thoughts and notes.*</u>

Meditation 49

Happiness makes up in height for what it lacks in length."

Robert Frost, American poet (1874-1963)

 Happiness is a high that can be fleeting, or it can last an hour or more. I've never 'done drugs '(I've never needed them) so I can only imagine the kind of high they offer. It seems like they only offer an escape from life. Happiness gives you the joy of being alive! As Robert Frost so eloquently puts it, the highs more than make up for the length of those happy moments.

<u>*Your thoughts and notes.*</u>

Meditation 50

"There is only one happiness in life, to love and be loved."

I don't totally agree with this statement. There are many kinds of happiness. I do agree with the part that says 'to love and be loved' is true happiness. It's a different kind of happiness that matures over a lifetime. You become happy that you have someone to love and respect. You are happy that, even in the bad times there is always someone there who can offer you a safe haven.
 So, while I don't totally agree, I still agree. What does it mean to you?

<u>*Your thoughts and notes.*</u>

Meditation 51

"Happiness is a how, not a what; a talent, not an object."

You can't find happiness.
But you can achieve it!
Think about that!

<u>*Your thoughts and notes.*</u>

Meditation 52

"Man enjoys the happiness he feels, woman the happiness she gives."

 I meditated on this point for a time.

I came to realise it notes one of the big differences between Men and Women.

Women are essentially nurturers who offer love and care and companionship and happiness.

Men are still the primeval hunters and empire builders. Having said that, many men are in touch with their feminine side and vice versa.

How about you?

<u>*Your thoughts and notes.*</u>

Meditation 53

Happiness is a warm puppy."

Charles M. Schulz, American cartoonist (1922-2000)

Can it really be that simple?

Sometimes it can…….

………. If you let it!

Final thoughts

Meditation will open up your creative thought patterns.

Use the meditations above, whenever life is going through a slightly down period. The inner feelings it will show you will always be a revelation to where your mind is at.

As a last thought, start a 'dream diary'.

When you open up your mind and allow it to become the creative wonder that it can be, you will find your dreams will become more vivid. Keep your dream diary next to your bed and write in it when you first wake up. Don't worry if you can't remember all the dreams, at first. After a while you will find the dreams take up a pattern. Maybe they will tell you something. Maybe the 'universal force', or whatever you wish to call it, is trying to tell you something.

What it is telling you is up to you to think about.

Perhaps you could meditate on it?